The Body Keeps the Score

This WookBook Belongs To

....

....

....

ISBN: 978-1-951161-95-8

Copyright © 2020 by TIMELINE Publishers

Note: This is an Unofficial Workbook of The Body Keeps The Score Designed to Enrich Your Reading Experience.

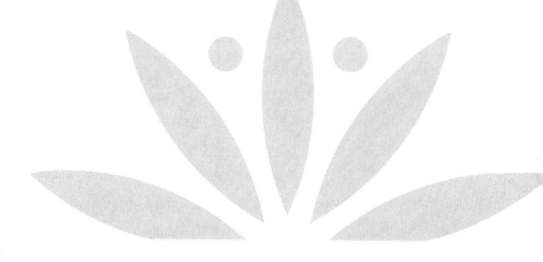

How to Use This Workbook To Achieve Your Goals

Complete beginners can begin using this Workbook for The Body Keeps The Score By Bessel van der Kolk.

The goal of this Workbook/Journal is to help even the newest readers to Start applying major lessons from The Book. Results have shown that Practicing the Things you're Grateful for each day will help you achieve your goals.

By using this Workbook, readers will find Awesome and Life-changing quotes by Bessel van der Kolk that we believed Played a Major role in defining the crucial messages of the author in the book.

There are Spaces for Personal Reflections, How You feel about a chapter (s) , also Space to Jot Down Lessons Learnt, Goals and Things you are grateful For. Take out a pencil, pen, or whatever digital technology you would put to use to jot down, implement, and make happen.

And don't forget to have fun - While at it. **This Workbook will help** you Discover the tremendous power of our relationships both to hurt and to heal—and offers new hope for reclaiming lives.

"

As long as you keep secrets
and suppress information,
you are fundamentally
at war with yourself···
The critical issue is allowing
yourself to know what
you know.
That takes an enormous
amount of courage.

Bessel A. van der Kolk

Personal Reflection

How This Chapter(s) Made Me Feel

Lessons Learnt

Lessons From Chapter (s)

_____
_____
_____
_____
_____
_____
_____
_____

Goals For Today

_____
_____
_____
_____
_____
_____
_____
_____

I am Grateful For...

_____
_____
_____
_____
_____
_____
_____
_____
_____
_____

Doodle

Note

Personal Reflection

How This Chapter(s) Made Me Feel

Lessons Learnt

Lessons From Chapter (s)

_____
_____
_____
_____
_____
_____
_____
_____
_____

Goals For Today

_____
_____
_____
_____
_____
_____
_____
_____
_____

I am Grateful For...

_____
_____
_____
_____
_____
_____
_____
_____
_____
_____

Doodle

"

Traumatized people chronically feel unsafe inside their bodies: The past is alive in the form of gnawing interior discomfort. Their bodies are constantly bombarded by visceral warning signs, and, in an attempt to control these processes, they often become expert at ignoring their gut feelings and in numbing awareness of what is played out inside. They learn to hide from their selves.

Bessel A. van der Kolk

Note

Personal Reflection

How This Chapter(s) Made Me Feel

Lessons Learnt

Lessons From Chapter (s)

_____
_____
_____
_____
_____
_____
_____
_____

Goals For Today

_____
_____
_____
_____
_____
_____
_____
_____

I am Grateful For...

_____
_____
_____
_____
_____
_____
_____
_____
_____
_____
_____

Doodle

Note

Personal Reflection

How This Chapter(s) Made Me Feel

Lessons Learnt

Lessons From Chapter (s)

Goals For Today

I am Grateful For...

Doodle

Note

"

Being able to feel safe with other people is probably the single most important aspect of mental health; safe connections are fundamental to meaningful and satisfying lives.

Bessel A. van der Kolk

Personal Reflection

_____
_____
_____
_____
_____
_____

How This Chapter(s) Made Me Feel

_____
_____
_____
_____
_____
_____
_____
_____
_____
_____

Lessons Learnt

Lessons From Chapter (s)

_____
_____
_____
_____
_____
_____
_____
_____

Goals For Today

_____
_____
_____
_____
_____
_____
_____

I am Grateful For...

_____
_____
_____
_____
_____
_____
_____
_____
_____
_____

Doodle

Note

Personal Reflection

_____

_____

_____

_____

_____

How This Chapter(s) Made Me Feel

_____

_____

_____

_____

_____

_____

_____

_____

_____

Lessons Learnt

Lessons From Chapter (s)

_____
_____
_____
_____
_____
_____
_____
_____
_____
_____

Goals For Today

_____
_____
_____
_____
_____
_____
_____
_____
_____
_____

I am Grateful For...

_____
_____
_____
_____
_____
_____
_____
_____
_____
_____
_____
_____

Doodle

"

As I often tell my students,
the two most important
phrases in therapy,
as in yoga, are
"Notice that" and
"What happens next?"
Once you start approaching
your body with curiosity
rather than with fear,
everything shifts.

Bessel A. van der Kolk

Note

Personal Reflection

_____

_____

_____

_____

_____

How This Chapter(s) Made Me Feel

_____

_____

_____

_____

_____

_____

_____

_____

_____

Lessons Learnt

Lessons From Chapter (s)

_____
_____
_____
_____
_____
_____
_____
_____

Goals For Today

_____
_____
_____
_____
_____
_____
_____
_____

I am Grateful For...

_____
_____
_____
_____
_____
_____
_____
_____
_____
_____
_____

Doodle

Note

Personal Reflection

How This Chapter(s) Made Me Feel

Lessons Learnt

Lessons From Chapter (s)

_____
_____
_____
_____
_____
_____
_____
_____
_____

Goals For Today

_____
_____
_____
_____
_____
_____
_____
_____
_____

I am Grateful For...

_____
_____
_____
_____
_____
_____
_____
_____
_____
_____
_____
_____

Doodle

Note

" Neuroscience research shows that the only way we can change the way we feel is by becoming aware of our inner experience and learning to befriend what is going inside ourselves.

Bessel A. van der Kolk

Personal Reflection

How This Chapter(s) Made Me Feel

Lessons Learnt

Lessons From Chapter (s)

Goals For Today

I am Grateful For...

Doodle

Note

Personal Reflection

How This Chapter(s) Made Me Feel

Lessons Learnt

Lessons From Chapter (s)	Goals For Today

I am Grateful For...

Doodle

66

Being traumatized means continuing to organize your life as if the trauma were still going on—unchanged and immutable—as every new encounter or event is contaminated by the past.

Bessel A. van der Kolk

Note

Personal Reflection

_____

_____

_____

_____

_____

How This Chapter(s) Made Me Feel

_____

_____

_____

_____

_____

_____

_____

_____

Lessons Learnt

Lessons From Chapter (s)

_____
_____
_____
_____
_____
_____
_____
_____

Goals For Today

_____
_____
_____
_____
_____
_____
_____
_____

I am Grateful For...

_____
_____
_____
_____
_____
_____
_____
_____
_____
_____

Doodle

Note

Personal Reflection

How This Chapter(s) Made Me Feel

Lessons Learnt

Lessons From Chapter (s)

_____
_____
_____
_____
_____
_____
_____
_____

Goals For Today

_____
_____
_____
_____
_____
_____
_____
_____

I am Grateful For...

_____
_____
_____
_____
_____
_____
_____
_____
_____
_____

Doodle

Note

"

As the ACE study has shown, child abuse and neglect is the single most preventable cause of mental illness, the single most common cause of drug and alcohol abuse, and a significant contributor to leading causes of death such as diabetes, heart disease, cancer, stroke, and suicide.

Bessel A. van der Kolk

Personal Reflection

How This Chapter(s) Made Me Feel

Lessons Learnt

Lessons From Chapter (s)

_____
_____
_____
_____
_____
_____
_____
_____
_____
_____

Goals For Today

_____
_____
_____
_____
_____
_____
_____
_____
_____
_____

I am Grateful For...

_____
_____
_____
_____
_____
_____
_____
_____
_____
_____
_____
_____

Doodle

Note

Personal Reflection

How This Chapter(s) Made Me Feel

Lessons Learnt

Lessons From Chapter (s)

_____
_____
_____
_____
_____
_____
_____
_____
_____
_____

Goals For Today

_____
_____
_____
_____
_____
_____
_____
_____
_____

I am Grateful For...

_____
_____
_____
_____
_____
_____
_____
_____
_____
_____
_____
_____

Doodle

Mindfulness not only makes it possible to survey our internal landscape with compassion and curiosity but can also actively steer us in the right direction for self-care.

Bessel A. van der Kolk

Note

Personal Reflection

_____

_____

_____

_____

_____

How This Chapter(s) Made Me Feel

_____

_____

_____

_____

_____

_____

_____

_____

_____

Lessons Learnt

Lessons From Chapter (s)

_____
_____
_____
_____
_____
_____
_____
_____

Goals For Today

_____
_____
_____
_____
_____
_____
_____
_____

I am Grateful For...

_____
_____
_____
_____
_____
_____
_____
_____
_____
_____

Doodle

Note

Personal Reflection

How This Chapter(s) Made Me Feel

Lessons Learnt

Lessons From Chapter (s)

_____
_____
_____
_____
_____
_____
_____
_____
_____
_____

Goals For Today

_____
_____
_____
_____
_____
_____
_____
_____
_____

I am Grateful For...

_____
_____
_____
_____
_____
_____
_____
_____
_____
_____
_____

Doodle

Note

66

One day he told me that he'd spent his adulthood trying to let go of his past, and he remarked how ironic it was that he had to get closer to it in order to let it go.

Bessel A. van der Kolk

Personal Reflection

How This Chapter(s) Made Me Feel

Lessons Learnt

Lessons From Chapter (s)

_____
_____
_____
_____
_____
_____
_____
_____
_____

Goals For Today

_____
_____
_____
_____
_____
_____
_____
_____

I am Grateful For...

_____
_____
_____
_____
_____
_____
_____
_____
_____
_____
_____

Doodle

Note

Personal Reflection

How This Chapter(s) Made Me Feel

Lessons Learnt

Lessons From Chapter (s)

_____
_____
_____
_____
_____
_____
_____
_____

Goals For Today

_____
_____
_____
_____
_____
_____
_____
_____

I am Grateful For...

_____
_____
_____
_____
_____
_____
_____
_____
_____
_____

Doodle

Note

Personal Reflection

_____
_____
_____
_____
_____

How This Chapter(s) Made Me Feel

_____
_____
_____
_____
_____
_____
_____
_____
_____

Lessons Learnt

Lessons From Chapter (s)

_____
_____
_____
_____
_____
_____
_____

Goals For Today

_____
_____
_____
_____
_____
_____
_____

I am Grateful For...

_____
_____
_____
_____
_____
_____
_____
_____
_____
_____

Doodle

"

It takes enormous trust and courage to allow yourself to remember.

Bessel A. van der Kolk

Note

Personal Reflection

How This Chapter(s) Made Me Feel

Lessons Learnt

Lessons From Chapter (s)

_____
_____
_____
_____
_____
_____
_____
_____

Goals For Today

_____
_____
_____
_____
_____
_____
_____
_____

I am Grateful For...

_____
_____
_____
_____
_____
_____
_____
_____
_____
_____

Doodle

Note

Personal Reflection

_____
_____
_____
_____
_____
_____

How This Chapter(s) Made Me Feel

_____
_____
_____
_____
_____
_____
_____
_____
_____
_____

Lessons Learnt

Lessons From Chapter (s)

_____
_____
_____
_____
_____
_____
_____
_____
_____

Goals For Today

_____
_____
_____
_____
_____
_____
_____
_____

I am Grateful For...

_____
_____
_____
_____
_____
_____
_____
_____
_____
_____

Doodle

Note

Note

Personal Reflection

How This Chapter(s) Made Me Feel

Lessons Learnt

Lessons From Chapter (s)

_____
_____
_____
_____
_____
_____
_____
_____
_____
_____

Goals For Today

_____
_____
_____
_____
_____
_____
_____
_____
_____
_____

I am Grateful For...

_____
_____
_____
_____
_____
_____
_____
_____
_____
_____
_____
_____

Doodle

Note

Personal Reflection

_____

_____

_____

_____

_____

_____

How This Chapter(s) Made Me Feel

_____

_____

_____

_____

_____

_____

_____

_____

_____

Lessons Learnt

Lessons From Chapter (s)

_____
_____
_____
_____
_____
_____
_____
_____

Goals For Today

_____
_____
_____
_____
_____
_____
_____
_____

I am Grateful For...

_____
_____
_____
_____
_____
_____
_____
_____
_____
_____
_____

Doodle

Note

Note

Thanks

We Congratulate you for taking that ultimate decision
And buying this Workbook, we hope you'll achieve
All Your Goals this New Year. You Got This!
Take out a little of your Time To Rate Us on Amazon.

Also we appreciate you for believing in Us and Buying this Workbook. May all Your Goals Actualize this Year!

Other Books By Same Author

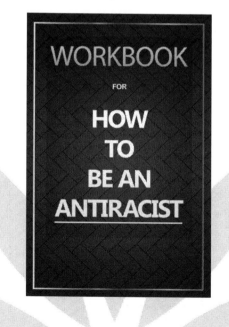

Manufactured by Amazon.ca
Bolton, ON